Flexible Dieting and IIFYM Cookbook

31 High Protein Recipes to Help You Lose Fat and Build Muscle

Table of Contents

Introduction

Hello, reader, and welcome to "Flexible Dieting and "If It Fits Your Macros" Cookbook: 31 High Protein Recipes to Help You Lose Fat and Build Muscle." This collection of recipes is designed and compiled to help you make the most out of your flexible diet as well as give you a wide variety of different foods to keep your eating habits not only healthy, but delicious as well.

With each recipe, you'll not only find the ingredients and step by step instructions, but you will also find the proper serving size and calories per serving to make sure you get all the information you need before diving into any one of these delectable dishes.

I would like to thank each and every one of you who picked this book up. I hope you enjoy every last one of the recipes in this book and share them with your friends and family.

Chapter 1: Breakfast

The problems with so many common breakfast foods that most people pick up from grocery stores are twofold: The food may either be unhealthy and won't fit into your flexible dieting plan, or if the foods do fit into your plan, they may not fill you up as much as you'd hoped. Both of these can become serious issues (especially if you face the same problem day after day) and can lead you to break away from your daily routine.

You don't have to worry any longer, readers! I've done the research and experimentation for you and have formed this comprehensive list of recipes to help you stay within your dietary limits while filling you up.

Recipe 1: Eggs With an Extra Kick of Macros

Serving Size: ½ skillet (2 eggs)

Time you will need to prepare your ingredients: 15 minutes
Time you will need to cook any ingredients: 10 minutes
Total Time to prepare and cook the meal: 25 minutes

Nutritional Information for one serving:
- Total Cals: 353 calories
- Protein: 21.9 grams
- Fat: 17 grams
- Fiber: 11 grams
- Carbohydrates: 30 grams

Ingredients:
- 4 large eggs (preferably organic)
- ½ a small onion (diced)
  - I prefer sweet onions, but you can use white or red if you like the flavor of either more.
- 1 Cup yellow squash (cubed)
- ½ a bell pepper (diced)
  - Like the onions, the color you use is up to you (I like the orange peppers personally.)
- 2 Cups kale (destemmed and chopped)
- ½ Cup blueberries (preferably organic or wild)
- 1 ripe avocado (sliced)
- 1 Tablespoon coconut oil
- 1 clove of fresh garlic (chopped or minced)
  - Garlic is entirely optional. Some people like it, some people don't.
- Salt
- Pepper

Directions:

1. Clean all of your vegetables and cut them according to the recipe. The cutting styles listed with the appropriate ingredients above are designed to help each of the different vegetables cook the quickest and, therefore, the most even.
2. Place a large skillet on the stove and crank the heat to medium, then drop the coconut oil and let it heat up. After about 30 seconds or so, add your chopped or minced garlic to let its flavor soak up in the oil.
3. Throw in all of your prepped vegetables (your onion, squash, bell peppers, and kale). Sauté your mixture for roughly 6 minutes, or until tender. It's important that you keep your vegetables moving while they are in the skillet so they don't burn to the sides.
4. Once your vegetables get to the consistency you want (tender to the touch), add your blueberries and a bit of pepper and salt. You can adjust the amount of Pepper and salt as you see fit, but if this is your first time trying anything like this, I suggest start with a pinch and go from there.
5. Keep your mixture of vegetables moving for about another minute before adding your eggs right on top of it. Scramble your eggs into your vegetable mixture making sure everything is spread evenly throughout the dish.
6. Cook your dish until the eggs are fully cooked (anywhere from 30 seconds to a minute and a half depending on your stove top). It's best to just keep an eye on the eggs. Once you see there are no more uncooked portions, remove the skillet from the heat.
7. While your eggs and vegetables cool down for a moment, remove the outer skin from your avocado and remove the seed. Slice each half of the avocado long ways into 4 - 6 slices.
8. Separate your eggs and vegetable mixture into two even servings and place half of the sliced avocado on the side of either serving.

You may also find yourself getting three or even four servings out of this dish. If that is the case, you may simply multiply the above numbers by two and divide the numbers you get by however many servings you can get from this recipe. That will tell you how many calories and macros you are getting with your personal adjusted serving size.

Recipe 2: Protein-Packed Pancakes

Serving Size: 8 pancakes (they are pretty small pancakes)

Time you will need to prepare your ingredients: 5 minutes
Time you will need to cook any ingredients: 15 minutes
Total Time to prepare and cook the meal: 20 minutes

Nutritional Information for one serving:
- Total Cals: 30 calories
- Protein: 53 grams
- Fat: 1.5 grams
- Fiber: 2 grams
- Carbohydrates: 19 grams

Ingredients:
- 4 large egg whites (about ½ cup)
- 1 scoop vanilla whey protein
    - 1 scoop is roughly 30 grams.
- ½ cup Greek Yogurt (0 percent fat is preferred but not necessary)
- 1 Tablespoon of all purpose flour
- 1 teaspoon of vanilla extract
- 2 teaspoons of sugar (or an artificial sweetener of your choice)
- 1 teaspoon of baking soda

Directions:
1. In a large bowl, mix all purpose flour, vanilla whey protein, sugar, and baking soda) with a whisk or plastic spatula.
2. Slowly mix in the egg whites. Once those are even mixed in, add in your greek yogurt followed by your vanilla extract.
3. Mix all of your ingredients together until the texture is consistent and there are no lumps or water areas.
4. Place a medium skillet over medium heat. Use a non-stick pan to remove the necessity of butter, oil, or nonstick spray. Pour ⅛ of your batter into the center of your skillet and let cook. When the middle of the pancake begins to produce bubbles that pop, you are ready to flip!
5. Cook each pancake one at a time and be patient (it will pay off in the end). Place all of the pancakes on a plate and enjoy!

You can top the pancakes with the classic toppings (powdered sugar, syrup. Fruit, or whipped cream) but do so at your own risk. Adding any of the listed toppings or any others you can think of will increase the calories and other nutrients in the pancakes. While a little bit of powdered sugar isn't good for you, it can make your dish a bit sweeter (especially for those bad mornings where you need a bit of extra happiness).

Recipe 3: Omelette With Spinach and Onion

Serving Size: 1 Omelette

Time you will need to prepare your ingredients: 5 minutes
Time you will need to cook any ingredients: 10 minutes
Total Time to prepare and cook the meal: 15 minutes

Nutritional Information for one serving:
- Total Cals: 428 calories
- Protein: 26.7 grams
- Fat: 24 grams
- Fiber: 5.5 grams
- Carbohydrates: 24.5 grams

Ingredients:
- 3 large eggs (organic is always preferred)
- 2 Cups of fresh, raw spinach
- ½ onion
  - I prefer white onions for this recipe, but you may use red or sweet.
- 2 strips of fresh bacon
  - Never use the precooked or microwave bacon as it has preservatives which will not help you when dieting (flexible or otherwise).
  - For this, I substitute turkey bacon because of its lower fat content relative to pork bacon.
- ¼ teaspoon vegetable oil
  - You may also use olive oil, but vegetable oil is lighter and, personally, I prefer the flavor.
- Pepper and salt

Directions:

1. In a small to medium sized bowl, crack the eggs and whisk them together to form a consistent color and texture. Use a whisk for best results (you may also use a fork to get the same results with a bit of extra effort).
2. Chop your spinach to the size you want (smaller pieces means the spinach will be more evenly spread throughout your omelette), then dice the half of an onion you have.
3. Mix your newly chopped and diced vegetables into your eggs so that they are evenly dispersed throughout.
4. Place a medium skillet (preferably nonstick) over a stove set to medium high heat (too hot and the edges of the omelette will burn, not hot enough and your eggs will take too long to cook). Place the olive oil in the skillet and swirl it around so that it covers every part of the bottom of the pan.
5. Pour the egg and vegetable mixture into the skillet. At this point, you can add a teaspoon of water to give the eggs a fluffier texture. Once the eggs start to form bubbles on the top, flip your omelette over and cook the other side for roughly a minute and a half (cooking time for either side of your omelette will vary depending on the skillet you use and your stove top).
6. Slide your Omelette onto a plate and fold it over and place it to the side.
   a. If you want crispier edges on your omelette, turn the heat up a bit (do not crank it up to high to get crispier edges). Let the omelette cook for an additional twenty seconds or so to allow the edges a moment to become crispy.
   b. For this step, you should constantly check the edges and bottom of the omelette to make sure it's not getting too brown or burning).
7. In the same pan, place your strips of bacon (turkey or pork) and cook them until the texture you like. If you like chewier bacon, make sure each of the pieces is cooked through completely before eating.

8. Once your bacon is cooked, place it on the plate with your omelette and enjoy!

This may be obvious to some of you readers out there, but you're always encouraged to mix up the ingredients you place inside your omelettes. Try a different type of onion, of use bell peppers to add a nice crunch. Kale works well instead of spinach. Substitutions, additions, and removing ingredients to make the recipe your own is always a great way to keep your daily meals interesting and, when you spend time to find out the perfect mixture, more satisfying.

Recipe 4: Quick and Easy Greek Yogurt with Fruit and Granola

Serving Size: 1 bowl

Time you will need to prepare your ingredients: 5 minutes
Time you will need to cook any ingredients: N/A
Total Time to prepare and cook the meal: 5 minutes

Nutritional Information for one serving:
- Total Cals: 245 calories
- Protein: 47 grams
- Fat: 2.1 grams
- Fiber: 5.2 grams
- Carbohydrates: 11 grams

Ingredients:
- 1 Cup Greek Yogurt
    - For this recipe you can either use plain or vanilla for a more "universal" flavor to go with different fruits. Different flavors of greek yogurt have slightly different calories and macro counts, so keep an eye out for that.
    - 1 Cup is just above a single serving greek yogurt cup (which usually comes in 227 gram containers). If you want to use a single serving cup, you can still follow the instructions after this exactly and the dish will be perfectly fine.
- 2 Tablespoons of granola
- 1 Banana sliced
    - I prefer to slice my bananas as thin as I can for this recipe to mix well with the greek yogurt while still staying relatively solid and banana textured.
- I 30 gram scoop of Vanilla whey protein.

Directions:
1. Move the yogurt to a bowl (do this even if you are using a single serving cup because you will need the extra space for the other ingredients).
2. Mix the scoop of vanilla whey protein so that it is evenly spread throughout the greek yogurt (you don't want any lumps or whey protein deposits that you can accidently bite into).
3. Slowly pour the granola of your choice into your yogurt and mix it so that all of the granola is covered with yogurt (the granola and yogurt don't need to be mixed nearly as much as the protein powder, so don't worry if there are clumps).
4. Finally, add the banana and gently stir the whole mixture so that the banana slices blend with the yogurt and granola. The faster and more aggressively you mix the banana slices in, the higher the risk of smashing the banana slices and giving them a more yogurt like texture. If you want the banana slices to blend, go to town. This part is entirely up to you.

This recipe is nice to have around because of how easy it is. It's quick to make and requires no cooking. You can always throw all of the ingredients together into a tupperware container (without mixing) and throw it sealed into your bag or backpack and let your daily motions do all the mixing for you! (You may want to give the mixture a good stir when you open it after your walking around, but walking should do a pretty decent job at mixing everything together.

Recipe 5: French Toast with a Kick

Serving Size: 3 slices of bread

Time you will need to prepare your ingredients: 5 minutes
Time you will need to cook any ingredients: 20 minutes
Total Time to prepare and cook the meal: 25 minutes

Nutritional Information for one serving:
- Total Cals: 300 calories
- Protein: 33 grams
- Fat: 10 grams
- Fiber: 4 grams
- Carbohydrates: 38 grams

Ingredients:
- 8 slices of low calorie bread
- ¾ cups milk
  - Although skim or 1 percent milk has few calories and macro counts, you really want that creamy texture. 2 percent milk, although a bit fattier, offers the perfect texture and thickness for your mixture.
- 3 large eggs (separate the yolk from the white in 1 of the eggs)
- 1 scoop vanilla whey protein powder (roughly 30 grams)
- Vanilla Extract
- A pinch of ground cinnamon
  - Freshly ground cinnamon sticks will always have a more potent and fresher flavor. If you have cinnamon sticks around the house, I suggest you use them, but pre ground cinnamon works as well.

Directions:
1. Set your oven's dial for 350 degrees Fahrenheit and set the bread aside.
2. Whisk together the milk and your 2 large eggs into a large mixing bowl. Once combined, slowly mix in the egg white until fully combined.
3. As you whisk, slowly add your scoop of vanilla whey protein powder until fully combined.
4. Pour a few drops of vanilla extract into the bowl.
   a. If you are using vanilla extract substitute (not pure vanilla extract) then feel free to add a bit more as pure vanilla extract is much more potent).
5. Finally, add your last ingredient: A pinch of ground cinnamon.
   a. If you really want to taste the cinnamon in your french toast, feel free to add more. However, be cautious, because an additional pinch will go a long way.
6. Dip each piece of bread into your mixture (one at a time) and place on a cookie sheet that has been coated in either oil or nonstick spray (you may require 2 baking sheets).
7. Once all 8 pieces of bread have been soaked in the mixture and placed on the oiled baking sheet, slide it onto a rack in your oven and set an alarm for 10 minutes.
8. After that 10 minutes is up, pull the baking sheet out of the over and, using a spatula or turner, flip each of the pieces of bread over.
9. Return the baking sheet to the over and set a second timer for another 10 minutes.
10. After the timer goes off, pull your french toast out of the oven and serve!

In terms of preparations, this meal is as easy as they come. This means there's lots of room for fiddling with the recipe and making it your own. The only thing keeping this recipe from being a great quick morning routine is the cook time and the break halfway through to flip your food. This is a pretty good recipe for any morning you have half an hour or so, but won't make a good recipe for baking while doing other chores or preparing for the day.

Recipe 6: Save-It-For-Later Sausage, Egg, and Cheese Sandwich

Serving Size: 1 Sandwich

Time you will need to prepare your ingredients: 5 minutes
Time you will need to cook any ingredients: 15 minutes
Tctal Time to prepare and cook the meal: 20 minutes

Nutritional Information for one serving:
- Total Cals: 264 calories
- Protein: 21 grams
- Fat: 8 grams
- Fiber: 8 grams
- Carbohydrates: 30 grams

Ingredients:
- 6 english muffins
- ½ pound of ground turkey sausage meat
- 6 slices of low fat cheddar cheese slices
- 6 large eggs
- Pepper and salt

Directions:
1. There are a few different ways you can prepare your eggs to best make them fit onto the english muffins, I'll list a few and you can decide which is easiest for you.
   a. Bake them in a muffin tin: Set your oven's dial to to 375 degrees Fahrenheit and grease a muffin tin liberally with oil or nonstick spray. Crack an egg into a cup and whisk with a fork until combined. Pour the mixed egg into one of the compartments of the muffin tin. Do this for all the eggs. Bake the eggs for 15 minutes (or until fully cooked).
   b. Cook them in a skillet (this one works best if you have a metal circular egg ring): Crack an egg into a cup and

whisk it together with a fork (just like in the baking method). Place a skillet onto your stove and set it to low heat. Once it's heated up, place your egg ring onto the flat part of the skillet and spray it with a spritz of nonstick spray (if you have multiple egg rings and are using a larger skillet, you can easily make several eggs at once using this method). Cook the eggs thoroughly (don't flip or turn the eggs. The low heat will cook them through without burning). Once cooked, use a turner or spatula to move the egg disks either onto a plate, or directly onto one of the english muffins.

2. In a skillet, cook your turkey sausage over medium-to-medium high heat. As each sausage finishes cooking, move it to a plate on the side, lined with paper towels to absorb any excess fat.

3. Once both the eggs and sausages are cooked, place one of each on each of your six english muffins and place a slice of low fat cheddar cheese on top. Add Pepper and salt until it tastes right to you.

4. You can either eat your sandwiches when they are ready, or you can place each in its own plastic bag or plastic wrap to freeze for up to two weeks.

To reheat your sausage, egg, and cheese english muffins:
1. Remove the frozen sandwich from the freezer.
2. Unwrap the sandwich from the cling wrap (or take out of the plastic bag) and rewrap in a paper towel.
3. Place a serving on a microwave safe plate and stick in the microwave for a minute to a minute and a half. Remove the sandwich, and enjoy!)

I highly recommend this recipe to anyone who has ever been, or has the chance to wake up late some mornings and need to grab something quick on the way out. The fact that you can freeze them for so long and stick them in the microwave, makes for an incredibly easy and quick breakfast, lunch, snack, or even dinner.

Chapter 2: Lunch

Lunch is easily the most flexible of the three main meals in a day. Of course, you can always eat pancakes for dinner or pizza for breakfast, but usually people stick to the norms for those meals. Lunch, however, can consist of pizza, or an omelette, or any other food that you can enjoy at anytime of the day without you getting too many weird looks.

The one shortcoming of lunch comes with having a job or responsibilities throughout the day. A nine-to-five job can put a pretty large wrench in any plans to have a wide variety of lunches while avoiding going out to eat everyday during your lunch break or breaking any diet habits you've picked up. So what is one to do to keep lunch tasty, healthy, and fun? I have several relatively easy meals that will not only fill you up, but will make your friends' and coworkers' mouths water from across the room.

Recipe 7: Chicken Burrito Bowl

Serving Size: 1 Bowl (half of the food prepared)

Time you will need to prepare your ingredients: 30 minutes
Time you will need to cook any ingredients: 20 minutes
Total Time to prepare and cook the meal: 50 minutes

Nutritional Information for one serving:
- Total Cals: 565 calories
- Protein: 55 grams
- Fat: 10 grams
- Fiber: 23 grams
- Carbohydrates: 67 grams

Ingredients:
- 2 Cups of rice
  - I use white rice for this recipe, but brown rice is also acceptable (switching will change your calorie and fiber amounts, though)
- 1 large lime
- 1 chicken breast (roughly 12 ounces)
- ⅓ cup black beans
  - Pick up the "no salt added" variety if you can.
- ½ cup of your favorite salsa brand
  - Because homemade is always better, I've include steps to making your own salsa at home. Not only does it taste better, but you get to make it just the way you like it.
- ¼ cup of guacamole
- ¼ cup 0% greek yogurt
- ¼ cup cheddar cheese
  - Like most things, getting fresh cheese is preferred, or at least blocks of cheese to shred yourself. If you can't find either, pre shredded cheese will work fine.
- 1 cup lettuce
- 1 lime

- ○ If you happen to have some lime juice lying around (some of the nicer stuff) then you may also use that. Fresh lime juice is always better, but can be messy.
- 3 teaspoons of fresh cilantro
- Your favorite Mexican seasoning (homemade or store bought will work equally well in this recipe)

Directions:
1. Chop your cilantro and lettuce. If it's necessary, shred your cheese at this point too. Cut your lime into four equal slices and set to the side.
2. Cook your rice in either a rice cooker or on the stove top.
3. Once your rice is cooked, toss it with your chopped cilantro and a pinch of salt. Once those are mixed, take ¼ of your lime and squeeze the juice into the rice mixture. Mix again until everything is well combined.
4. Toss your chicken breasts with the Mexican seasoning and cook.
    a. You may grill or bake your chicken as you desire.
5. When the chicken is cooked through, cut it into small bite-sized pieces (about ½ inch).
    a. You may also cut your chicken before seasoning and cooking. This will allow for a more even coat of seasoning (which will require a bit more seasoning) as well as a faster cooking time.
6. In a large bowl (one safe for the microwave), pour your beans. Microwave them for 30 seconds. Be sure to stir the beans a few times and place them back in the microwave for another 15 seconds each time. Do this until the beans have a consistent warmth throughout. That's the end of the cooking!

Building your Bowl:
1. Place out two bowls, side by side.
   a. You can buy bowls similar to the disposable ones they use at Chipotle restaurants, but I find it to be much easier, convenient, and better for the environment if you place the chicken and other ingredients into tupperware or a higher end lunch box directly.
2. Divide the ingredients evenly between your two containers. (this is my preferred order, but you can do it in any order you wish).
   a. Rice
   b. Seasoned chicken breast
   c. Black beans
   d. Salsa
   e. Guacamole
   f. Greek yogurt
   g. Shredded cheese
   h. Chopped lettuce
3. Add one of the slices of lime on the side if you so desire for that extra squirt of citrus when you eat it later.

Salsa Directions:
Ingredients:
- 3 medium tomatoes
- 1 onion
  - I prefer red for salsa, but this is always up to you.
- 1 jalapeno pepper
- 1 lime (or 1 ½ Tablespoon of lime juice)
- ½ cup cilantro
- Pepper and salt

Directions:
1. Dice the tomatoes and the onion. You may cut them to be slightly large cubes (¼ inch) or smaller for a more consistent texture. Cut the jalapeno pepper into small cubes as well (dice it, but finer than you would your tomatoes and onions. This is called a Brunoise dice).
    a. Be careful with the onions and jalapeno peppers, especially after you cut them. The juices can get everywhere and will definitely be on your fingers. Using disposable gloves can help prevent accidental eye rubs (if only to serve as a reminder not to do it).
    b. The seed of the jalapeno pepper are what add heat. If you want less heat, don't add the seeds or take the pepper out altogether. If you want more heat, add more seeds.
2. Add your cut foods to a medium sized bowl and add your lime juice, cut cilantro, and a pinch of both Pepper and salt. Mix the ingredients together and there's your homemade salsa!

If you like the idea of this recipe, but don't like chicken so much, you can always swap out your protein for something else. Steak and tofu can be great substitutions. You can even remove or add ingredients as you see fit (of course, while keeping track of the calorie and macro additions or subtractions as well). Sour cream, different kinds of cheeses, brown rice, different meats, different peppers or even chillies will change the flavor of your burrito bowl and salsa drastically. Play around with it and find the recipe that best first both your taste preference and your daily allotted calories and macro counts.

Recipe 8: Flexible Slow cooker Chicken Tortilla Soup

Serving Size: 1 bowl

Time you will need to prepare your ingredients: 20 minutes
Time you will need to cook any ingredients: 6 hours
Total Time to prepare and cook the meal: 6 hours 20 minutes

Nutritional Information for one serving:
- Total Cals: 218 calories
- Protein: 32 grams
- Fat: 6 grams
- Fiber: 9 grams
- Carbohydrates: 31 grams

Ingredients:
- 10 ounces of enchilada sauce
- 10 ounces of corn off the cob
- 10 ounces kidney beans
- Four ounces green chiles
- 1 large tomato
- 2 Tablespoons of lime juice
- 1 chicken breast (roughly 12 ounces)
- ½ ounce of Ranch seasoning mix (roughly ½ of a packet)
- 2 cups of cilantro
- 1 onion
    - I prefer white for this recipe
- 1 clove of garlic
- ½ Tablespoon of olive oil
- 1 teaspoon chili powder
- 1 teaspoon cumin
- 4 chicken bouillon cubes
- 1 Cup salsa (you can use the simple homemade recipe I provided with the last recipe!)
- 2 Cups water

Directions:

1. Dice your tomato and onion (but keep them separate). Mince your garlic, chop your cilantro, and dice your green chile.
   a. You can cut these all when they are required to go into the soup, but it's easier to just get the cutting out of the way first.
2. In a pan, add olive oil, bouillon cubes, and your diced onion. Set on medium high heat and stir constantly until the onions are sweated and become brown.
3. Move your mixture to a large slow cooker and add your enchilada sauce, corn, beans, chiles, tomato, lime juice, Ranch seasoning, cumin, chili powder, salsa, chicken breast, water, and half of your cilantro.
4. Set the slow cooker on high and close and ignore for 6 hours.
5. Once the chicken is cooked through, take it out and place is in a bowl or on a large cutting board. Use two forks to pull the meat apart then return it to your slow cooker.
6. Switch your slow cooker to its "keep warm" setting and serve.
7. Sprinkle cilantro on top of each bowl.
8. You can serve the soup directly from the slow cooker fresh, place in the refrigerator for up to half a week, or freeze it for up to a quarter year.

If you want a bit more to your soup, you can add tortilla chips, cheese, or sour cream on top after it's been heated or reheated. Keep track of the calories and macros in each additional topping, because they can add a lot.

Recipe 9: Chicken and Cheese Potatoes

Serving Size: 1 ½ Cups (Makes 4 servings)

Time you will need to prepare your ingredients: 10 minutes
Time you will need to cook any ingredients: 55 minutes
Total Time to prepare and cook the meal: 1 hour and 5 minutes

Nutritional Information for one serving:
- Total Cals: 450 calories
- Protein: 28 grams
- Fat: 13 grams
- Fiber: 4 grams
- Carbohydrates: 32 grams

Ingredients:
- 1 chicken breast
- 1 large onion
  - This recipe works better with Sweet yellow or white onions (red onions don't work too well).
- 2 bell peppers
- ¼ Cup of mushrooms
- 2 potatoes
- 2 Tablespoons Olive oil
- 4 slices provolone cheese
  - You can use any brand you want (as long as you realize the differences in calories and macro counts). I prefer Boar's head brand, but that doesn't mean you have to use it by any means.
- Pepper and salt

Directions:
1. Set your oven's dial to 450 degrees Fahrenheit. Peel both potatoes and slice them thin.
2. In a medium mixing bowl, toss thin cut potatoes, olive oil, and a few pinches of pepper and salt. Toss them until the olive oil and salt cover all of the potatoes evenly.

3. Liberally spray a baking sheet down with olive oil or butter and set French fries in a single layer on it (it may take two baking sheets). Place the potato slices in the oven and set the timer for 20 to 40 minutes. Check on them every few minutes after 25 minutes or so and look for the signs the fries are finished (golden brown and crispy).
    a. If you want to make thicker cut french fries, set the timer for 45 minutes instead of 25. They will take longer to cook and will come out softer.
4. While the french fries bake, cut the chicken breast into small pieces (around a quarter of an inch thick). Throw those into an oiled skillet and cook until they lose their pink color (about 2 minutes).
5. Dice your onions and mushroom caps and cut your bell peppers into long, thin strips. Sauté the three ingredients in another well-oiled skillet until the onions are translucent.
6. In a large bowl, mix the cooked chicken breast and sautéed onions, bell peppers, and mushrooms until evenly combined.
7. Take one fourth of your mixture and place it back into a skillet. Place a single slice of cheese on top of the pile and let it sit for a minute (just so the cheese begins to melt). Once the cheese begins to drip, stir it into the chicken and vegetables. Once mixed, set aside and repeat with the other three servings.
8. Once the french fries are done baking, put one fourth of the fries (about ½ of a potato's worth) onto a plate and top with one of the servings of chicken breast and vegetables.

You can always use frozen french fries, hash browns, or tater tots to mix up the texture and consistency of the dish, but french fries are offer a nice long piece of potato to bite into. Add more cheese (or gravy) if you want a bit more flavor, but both affect the calories and macro counts relatively drastically.

Recipe 10: Protein Rich Cheesy Macaroni

Serving Size: 1 Cup (makes 8 servings)

Time you will need to prepare your ingredients: 5 minutes
Time you will need to cook any ingredients: 10 minutes
Total Time to prepare and cook the meal: 15 minutes

Nutritional Information for one serving:
- Total Cals: 310 calories
- Protein: 16 grams
- Fat: 8 grams
- Fiber: 3 grams
- Carbohydrates: 29 grams

Ingredients:
- 1 box (1 pound) of whole wheat noodles
  - In classic macaroni fashion, I suggest using elbow macaroni. But, understandably, not everyone is a fan of the noodle type. In this case, feel free to use any kind of noodle made to hold sauce (no spaghetti or angel hair). Be sure to cook the noodles accordingly.
- 2 Cups of sharp cheddar cheese
- 2 ½ cups milk
  - Like most recipes, 2% milk will offer a creamier cheese sauce, but skim or 1% contains less fat and calories. I suggest 1% for this particular recipe to have a nice mixture of creamy and calorie efficient.
- 3 Tablespoons all purpose flour
- 4 Tablespoons of fat free or light cream cheese

Directions:

1. Cook the elbow macaroni (or other noodle type) according to the box's instructions (usually boil around 9 to 12 minutes depending on the noodle and brand). Drain the noodles once cooked and set aside for later.
2. In a medium saucepan, mix flour and a couple of pinches of salt. Turn to medium heat and pour in the milk. Whisk the mixture as the saucepan heats up.
3. As the milk starts to boil, add the cream cheese and stir constantly.
4. Once it does reach a boil, reduce the heat to medium-low and let the mixture simmer for an additional couple of minutes. This will thicken the sauce to a nice consistency.
5. Remove the saucepan from the heat and pour your cheese over the mixture, stirring it in until the texture is consistent and all of the cheese is melted.
6. In a large bowl (or the pasta pot you used to cook the pasta) mix the noodles and cheese sauce until combined.

Recipe 11: Shellfish and Avocado Salad with Lime

Serving Size: 1 Cup (makes 4 servings)

Time you will need to prepare your ingredients: 20 minutes
Time you will need to cook any ingredients: 5 minutes*
Total Time to prepare and cook the meal: 25 minutes

Nutritional Information for one serving:
- Total Cals: 197 calories
- Protein: 25 grams
- Fat: 8 grams
- Fiber: 3 grams
- Carbohydrates: 7 grams

Ingredients:
- 1 pound shrimp (pre peeled to make things easier)*
  - Precooked shrimp, while not ideal, is much easier so don't be ashamed if you do not care to spend the effort cooking the shrimp yourself.
- 1 avocado
- 1 tomato
- ⅛ red onion
- I jalapeno
- 1 Tablespoon cilantro
- 1 teaspoon of olive oil
- 2 limes
  - You can substitute this with 3 ½ Tablespoons of lime juice.
- Pepper and salt

Directions:

1. If you're cooking the shrimp yourself, now would be the time to do that. I strongly suggest using higher end pre cooked shrimp because it makes it much easier and saves you a lot of time.
2. Prep your vegetables:
   a. Dice the onion so that you have roughly ¼ cups.
   b. Dice the tomato in the same way.
   c. Peel the avocado and remove the pit, then dice to ¼ - 12 inch cubes.
   d. Cut the jalapeno down the middle, remove the seeds and stem and dice.
   e. Chop cilantro into small pieces.
3. In a small mixing bowl, toss in your diced onion, olive oil, lime juice, and a pinch of Pepper and salt (you can always add more later) and cover with a paper towel. Set aside for at least 5 minutes.
4. Chop the cooked shrimp and, in a large mixing bowl, add the, jalapeno, avocado, tomato, and shrimp. Stir together so that everything is mixed well.
5. Scrape your onion, olive oil, lime juice, and Pepper and salt mixture into the large mixing bowl and stir until well combined. Add cilantro and mix so it's evenly spread throughout the dish.
6. Add more salt, pepper, or lime juice to fit your own taste.

*Cooking time only applies if you do not buy pre cooked shrimp.

Recipe 12: Zucchini Linguine

Ok, so it's not technically linguine, but it's hard to pass up such a nice sounding name for a recipe.

Serving Size: About 1 ½ cups of "pasta" (Makes 8 servings)

Time you will need to prepare your ingredients: 20 - 30 minutes
Time you will need to cook any ingredients: 40 minutes
Total Time to prepare and cook the meal: 60 - 70 minutes

Nutritional Information for one serving:
- Total Cals: 275 calories
- Protein: 26 grams
- Fat: 13 grams
- Fiber: 2.2 grams
- Carbohydrates: 13 grams

Ingredients:
- 1 pounds ground beef
  - Ground turkey makes a great substitute and will reduce the amount of calories and fat you ingest while eating this!
- ½ onion
- 1 28 ounce can of diced tomatoes
- 2 Tablespoons of basil
- 3 Zucchini
- 3 cloves of garlic
- 1 ½ cups of ricotta cheese
- ¼ cups of Parmigiano Reggiano cheese (the king of cheeses)
- 4 cups of shredded mozzarella cheese
- Olive oil
- Pepper and salt

"Noodle" Directions:
1. Peel the zucchini and slice it into thin, long strips (cut them into the shape of noodles)
2. Place the zucchini "noodles" onto a plate lined with paper towels and cover with salt. Wait 5 minutes and pat the zucchini dry.
3. Pour about half a teaspoon of olive oil into a skillet and turn it to medium low heat. Use a pair of tongs to place some of the zucchini noodles into the pan and cook until tender and limp (they should almost feel like cooked noodles).
4. Set aside for the time being.

Sauce Directions:
1. In a medium skillet, cook the beef until it reaches a nice brown color. Drain then return to the skillet. Mince the garlic and add it, your minced onions, and a Tablespoon of olive oil to the meat. Once the garlic begins to have a stronger smell (about 2 minutes) add tomatoes, freshly cut basil, and a pinch of both Pepper and salt. Stir to combine, then cover and turn the heat down to low. Simmer for half an hour to roughly 45 minutes.
2. About 5 minutes before your sauce is ready (30 - 35 minutes into cooking) add your ricotta and mozzarella cheese and stir to combine.
3. Once done, pour your zucchini noodles into the sauce and toss until the noodles are fully coated in sauce. Sprinkle parmigiano reggiano cheese on top and serve.

This is another fun recipe to try just because of how out of the ordinary it is. While the dish itself isn't too exciting or creative (it is essentially spaghetti, after all) the small adjustment to the noodles will have people slapping their foreheads and saying "now why didn't I think of that?"

Chapter 3: Dinner

Dinner is that one meal a day where you might get the whole family together to sit down and take a break from everyone's long and stressful day (in a perfect world, anyways). But, assuming your family does get together every now and again, you'll want to make foods that won't only keep them healthy, but will wow them in the process.

This chapter covers foods that are a bit heavier than breakfast foods (as well as some lunch foods) that will be sure to fill your family up for the entire night. People who go to bed full, after all, won't be tempted to sneak into the refrigerator at night for a midnight snack.

Recipe 13: Sweet Potatoes Stuffed With Buffalo Chicken

Serving Size: 1 Stuffed Potato

Time you will need to prepare your ingredients: 15 minutes
Time you will need to cook any ingredients: 1 hour
Total Time to prepare and cook the meal: 1 hour and fifteen minutes

Nutritional Information for one serving:
- Total Cals: 318 calories
- Protein: 30 grams
- Fat: 10.7 grams
- Fiber: 4 grams
- Carbohydrates: 25.2 grams

Ingredients:
- 7 sweet potatoes (medium sized)
- Two or three chicken breasts (they should be a combined measure of 30 ounces)
- 7 Tablespoon blue cheese or ranch dressing

Buffalo Sauce Ingredients:
- 1 ½ Tablespoon white vinegar
- ½ teaspoon Worcestershire sauce
- 1 clove fresh garlic
- 4 Tablespoons of unsalted butter
- 1 teaspoon cornstarch
- 1 Tablespoon of water
- ⅔ cups of hot sauce

Directions:
1. Set your oven's dial to to 400 degrees Fahrenheit. As that is warming up, line a baking sheet with aluminum foil (you may need two baking sheets) and place the seven potatoes on it. Make sure the potatoes aren't touching.

2. Once the oven is preheated, place your baking sheet (or multiple baking sheets) in and set a time for half an hour.
   a. When your potatoes are fully cooked, their skin and flesh will be tender and easy to cut with a knife.
3. Once the potatoes are done cooking, turn off the oven but leave the baking sheets in there to help keep the potatoes warm.
4. While the potatoes are baking, place the chicken breasts in a large pot. Pour water over them so no part sticks above the surface. Turn on your stove to high heat and let the chicken cook for half an hour.
5. In another pot (or the same one as the chicken if you want to wait for the meat to cook before moving on), combine hot sauce, vinegar, and Worcestershire sauce. Turn the stovetop's heat to low and mix.
6. While your sauce slowly heats up, mince the clove of garlic and throw it into the pot with the sauce. Next, add your butter to the sauce and increase the heat to medium. Mix continuously while the butter melts.
7. Once the butter is completely melted, add the cornstarch to the sauce and whisk for another 30 seconds to a minute until the sauce has thickened. Turn off the heat.
8. Remove the cooked chicken from its pot and shred it using two forks to pull the meat apart. Once shredded completely, add the chicken to your sauce and mix until the sauce fully covers the shredded chicken.
9. Finally, remove the sweet potatoes from the over and cut them almost in half (you want to create a hinge of sorts on the bottom so they don't slide apart). Stuff the sweet potatoes with your buffalo chicken and drizzle with blue cheese dressing or ranch dressing and server.

Of course, you don't have to use blue cheese dressing or ranch dressing at all. The recipe I have provided accounts for a light drizzle of one or the other, but removing them from the recipe would reduce the fat you ingest by a few points.

Recipe 14: Slow cooker Skinny Turkey Chili

Serving Size: 1 bowl (1 cup)

Time you will need to prepare your ingredients: 10 minutes
Time you will need to cook any ingredients: 6 hours
Total Time to prepare and cook the meal: 6 hours, 10 minutes

Nutritional Information for one serving:
- Total Cals: 254 calories
- Protein: 25 grams
- Fat: 6 grams
- Fiber: 9 grams
- Carbohydrates: 30 grams

Ingredients:
- 1 onion
- 1 pound of ground turkey
  - When it comes to meat, fresh is always better. If the town in which you live has a local butcher shop, go there first. You may pay a little more, but the fresh ground, never frozen meat will taste noticeably better.
- 1 16 ounce can of diced tomatoes
- 1 16 ounce can of red kidney beans (not flavored)
- 1 16 ounce can of chili beans (no salt added)
- 1 8 ounce can of green chiles
- ¼ Tablespoon of Cumin
- 1 ½ Tablespoon of Chili powder

  - The onion's color is up to you, as always, but I like sweet yellow onions in my chili.
  - The size also matters a bit for this recipe. A larger onion will mean a higher percent of your chili's body will be onion. I like a lot of onions, so I use large ones. If you like less onion, buy a smaller one.

Directions:
1. In a medium skillet, cook your turkey so it turns a nice brown hue (when it's cooked all the way through). Once the turkey has cooked out a bit of it's fat (yes there is fat, but since we're using turkey, it's a very little amount), dice your onion and throw that directly into the same skillet.
2. Throw your cooked turkey and onion mixture into your slow cooker. Drain and pour into the same slow cooker your chili beans and red kidney beans.
3. Without draining, empty your diced tomatoes and green chilis into the slow cooker.
4. Add your chili powder and cumin to your slow cooker and stir everything together.
5. Close the slow cooker and turn the temperature to low. Walk away and don't even think about it for 6 hours. When you return, you'll have a nice pot of chili ready for you!

Personally, I like my chili a bit spicier than most people like theirs. To check the flavor, I'll return to my crockpot every hour and a half or so, remove the top, and give the whole food a few sniffs. If it doesn't smell like I think it should, I'll sprinkle some more chili powder over it and maybe add some red pepper flakes.

Chili (especially slow cooker chili) is a great meal to experiment with. Even browsing through the spices you have in your cabinet can lead to some great if not weird combinations of flavors. Chili also freezes well for later eating (you can really save it for a rainy day).

Recipe 15: Spinach and Artichoke Casserole

Serving Size: Around 1 ½ cups (makes 16 servings)

Time you will need to prepare your ingredients: 10 minutes
Time you will need to cook any ingredients: 30 minutes
Total Time to prepare and cook the meal: 40 minutes

Nutritional Information for one serving:
- Total Cals: 183 calories
- Protein: 10 grams
- Fat: 9 grams
- Fiber: 0 grams
- Carbohydrates: 8 grams

Ingredients:
- 40 ounces of frozen spinach
  - You can usually fine these in packets of 10 ounces.
- 1 14 ounce can of artichoke hearts
- 1 cup of fat free sour cream
- 8 ounces of fat free cream cheese
- 2 ½ cups parmesan cheese
  - You will shred 2 cups of the parmesan cheese and grate the remaining ½ half cup.
- 4 cloves of garlic
- Pepper and salt

Directions:
1. The night before you plan to make a Spinach and Artichoke Casserole, thaw the frozen spinach in the refrigerator.
2. Set your oven's dial to to 375 degrees Fahrenheit.
3. Drain your now thawed spinach in a colander or strainer and chop it into small pieces. Drain the can of artichoke hearts and cut those into equally small pieces (try your best to match the size of the spinach -- consistency is key). Throw both ingredients into a large bowl and stir to combine.

4. Remove the skin from the cloves of garlic and mince. Place it in a small skillet and set the heat to medium. Let the garlic sweat for a few minutes until you can smell it from a few feet away.

5. While the garlic is sweating, grate 2 cups of the parmesan cheese (you can grate the other ½ cup now if you want, or save it for later if the garlic finished cooking).

6. In a bowl safe for microwave use, microwave the cream cheese 30 seconds. Stir it, and place it in the microwave again for an additional 15 seconds. If the cream cheese isn't soft (and fairly warm) repeat the process by placing the cream cheese back in the microwave for 10 second intervals.

7. Once soft, drop the cream cheese into the spinach and artichoke hearts and stir until the texture is consistent. If the cream cheese is soft enough, this shouldn't take much effort.

8. Drop the sour cream, grated parmesan cheese, and cooked garlic into the cream cheese mixture and stir until everything is combined. Add Pepper and salt to get the taste where you want it.

9. Into a casserole dish (or any other 9x11 oven safe baking dish) spoon your mixed ingredients. Cover the oven safe dish with aluminum foil and place into your oven. Bake for 20 to 25 minutes (depending on your oven).

10. At this point, your Spinach and Artichoke Casserole may seem close to finish, but it will be a bit soggy. Take the foil off the top and adjust the heat to 400 degrees Fahrenheit.

11. Continue baking at 400 degrees for an additional 8 minutes or until the edges begin to have a nice golden brown color and the top has a thin and crispy layer.

Many people aren't huge fans on spinach, but this recipe allows you to sneak in the nutrient rich plant into a meal without hardly anyone noticing. The cheese does well to cover up the taste and the artichoke hearts add a nice chewy texture to the whole thing.

Recipe 16: Healthy Fried Rice

Serving Size: 1 Cup (makes 4 servings)

Time you will need to prepare your ingredients: 5 minutes
Time you will need to cook any ingredients: 15 minutes
Total Time to prepare and cook the meal: 20 minutes

Nutritional Information for one serving:
- Total Cals: 245 calories
- Protein: 33 grams
- Fat: 5 grams
- Fiber: 2 grams
- Carbohydrates: 15 grams

Ingredients:
- 1 cup rice
  - You *can* use white rice for this, but brown rice is relatively full of nutrients and a lot of extra flavor.
- 2 chicken breasts (around 1 pound's worth)
  - You can switch the chicken out with another form of protein such as steak, shrimp, or tofu. If you do decide to do this, remember to adjust your numbers accordingly.
- 3 large egg (separate the yolks and whites from two of those eggs)
- ½ onion
- ¼ cup carrots
- ¼ cup peas
- 2 cloves of fresh garlic
  - You can use pre minced garlic, but fresh always offers a better flavor. It does take extra work, and can use an additional dish, but it's worth it.
- 2 Tablespoons of soy sauce
  - you can always add more soy sauce later for more flavor. You can do this during the cooking process or after while you are eating the dish. It's entirely up to you.

Directions:
1. Follow the instructions on the box or bag of rice to cook it fully.
   a. Many people use a rice cooker, a steamer, or boil the rice. I prefer to boil water, add rice, and let it soak the water up and cook off of heat.
2. While the rice cooks, cook the chicken breasts in a large skillet (be sure to use one you have a tight fitting lid for). Once cook, move to a cutting board and cube into small cubes (roughly twice the size of your peas).
3. Return the chicken to the skillet. Peel and mince your garlic and throw it into the skillet with your chicken. Turn the stove to medium low heat and let the garlic sweat while keeping the chicken moving so it doesn't burn.
4. Cut your carrots into small cubes (roughly the same size as the peas) and add both to the skillet with the chicken.
5. At this point, the rice should almost be done cooking. Remove it from the pan or steamer and place it into the skillet with everything else. Stir everything together. Add soy sauce and mix until the soy sauce isn't pooled anywhere. Pour ¼ cups of water into the skillet and mix.
6. Place the lid onto the skillet, turn the stove up to medium to medium high heat, and let sit for 3 - 5 minutes. Shake the skillet every minute or so to make sure the rice on the bottom doesn't burn.
7. Remove the lid from the skillet, mix the rice, and turn the stove back down to medium low heat. Let it sit for an additional 5 minutes to make sure all the water evaporates (you may want to mix once or twice in that time to prevent burning still), and serve!

Let's be honest, sometimes you just crave Chinese food. Most restaurants (especially the open buffet or the delivery restaurants) don't always carry the healthiest foods. You have to quench that hunger somehow, and this fried rice recipe will do just that!

Recipe 17: Bell Peppers Stuffed with Turkey and Cheese

Serving Size: 1 Stuffed pepper half (makes 6 servings)

Time you will need to prepare your ingredients: 15 minutes
Time you will need to cook any ingredients: 45 minutes
Total Time to prepare and cook the meal: 1 hour

Nutritional Information for one serving:
- Total Cals: 222 calories
- Protein: 18 grams
- Fat: 3 grams
- Fiber: 3.2 grams
- Carbohydrates: 19 grams

Ingredients:
- 1 pound of ground turkey meat
- 3 Bell peppers
- 1 clove of garlic
- ¼ of an onion
  - Sweet yellow onions work best for this recipe, white onions also work. Red onions will not mix well with the other flavors.
- 1 Tablespoon of cilantro
  - As usual, fresh is always better.
- 1 teaspoon cumin
- 1 Cup of chicken broth
- ¼ cup of tomato sauce
- 1 ½ Cus of brown rice
- 1 teaspoon garlic powder
- 6 Tablespoons of cheddar cheese
- Salt
- Olive oil

Directions:
1. Set your oven's dial to to 400 degrees Fahrenheit. Start cooking rice in any manner you are most comfortable.
2. In a small skillet, begin to brown your ground turkey.
3. Dice your onion, peel and mince your garlic, and cut your cilantro. Throw the three ingredients into medium sized skillet over medium heat with some olive oil. Sauté until the onions become translucent (around 2 ½ minutes).
4. Once your turkey is cooked, throw it in the other skillet with your onion, garlic, and cilantro. On top of that add garlic powder, cumin, and a pinch of salt. Stir to combine.
5. Next, add the tomato sauce and half of your chicken broth (½ cup). Mix everything together and turn the heat down to low. Allow the watery mixture to simmer for anywhere between 5 - 7 minutes.
6. Add your rice to the skillet and stir until combined. Let sit for a few minutes while the rice absorbs some of the excess broth.
7. While that finishes cooking, wash each of your bell peppers and cut into two equal halves. Remove the seeds and insides (to make a sort of bowl) and the stems from the tops. On a baking sheet, place each of the 6 halves of bell peppers onto it.
8. Scoop roughly one sixth of the turkey rice into each of the bell pepper halves and sprinkle each with a bit of cheese.
9. Pour the remaining ½ cup of chicken broth into the bottom of the baking sheet, cover the whole thing in more aluminum foil, and slide into the oven.
10. Bake for 40 - 45 minutes (depending on your oven it may take up to 55 minutes).
11. When the timer goes off, remove the sheet and carefully peel the aluminum foil from over your Bell Peppers Stuffed with Turkey and Cheese.

This recipe is a fun and creative way to present food elegantly. You can serve it with soup or salad on the side for a complete dining experience if you want. The one shortcoming of this recipe is the fact you can store the bell peppers in the fridge or freezer (they do not heat up well). Chances are you won't have leftovers to store though because these bell pepper bowls will go fast!

Recipe 18: Chicken Lo Mein

Serving Size: 1 ½ cups

Time you will need to prepare your ingredients: 20 minutes
Time you will need to cook any ingredients: 25 minutes
Total Time to prepare and cook the meal: 45 minutes

Nutritional Information for one serving:
- Total Cals: 355 calories
- Protein: 31 grams
- Fat: 4 grams
- Fiber: 3 grams
- Carbohydrates: 48 grams

Ingredients:
- 2 chicken breasts
  - The total combined weight of your chicken should be anywhere between 1 ½ pounds to around 2 pounds. Any more and you're calories and macro counts will be off from this recipe, and less and you'll hardly have any chicken at all!
- 1 16 ounce box of linguine
- 1 onion
- 4 carrots
- 4 cloves of garlic
- 1 ½ cups of green onions
- 1 teaspoon of garlic powder
- 1 teaspoon of cornstarch
- 4 cups of broth
  - For the broth, I suggest using either chicken or vegetable (do not use beef). The chicken broth will blend well with the ingredients (like the chicken) but the vegetable broth will add a nice variety of flavor.

Directions:

1. In a large skillet, cook the chicken through so that it is no longer pink. This can take anywhere from 5 minutes to around 7 ½ minutes depending on your stove (when in doubt, cook for longer).

2. As the chicken cooks, mince your four cloves of garlic and throw those in with the chicken. Make sure to mix it up so the garlic starts to cook.

3. Once the chicken is cooked through, slowly pour the broth directly over it and let it heat up (about a minute and a half).

4. In the meantime, take your box of linguine and cut the noodles in half. Drop the shortened noodles into the boiling broth and let boil for 3 - 4 minutes.

5. While the broth is boiling, dice your onion, green onion. Peel and slice your carrots into 2 inch pieces (or you can grate them if you like a finer texture). Throw your onion, green onions, carrot slices, soy sauce, garlic powder, and cornstarch into your boiling broth and stir until combined.

6. Reduce the heat to a simmer (medium to medium low) and let cook for 10 to 15 minutes. Every 3 minutes or so, give the mixture a stir to keep things cooking evenly.

If you find your broth boiling off too quickly, feel free to add more to balance it (if anything, you'll need to give your lo mein an additional minute or two to boil off any excess your pour in).

Chapter 4: Desserts

What can be said about desserts other than the obvious? Sure, you could grab a candy bar or a bowl of ice cream to help satisfy your sweet tooth, or you can enjoy one of these fantastic and healthy alternatives to keep you losing weight.

Recipe 19: Protein Rice Krispies Treats

Serving Size: 1 Bar

Time you will need to prepare your ingredients: 10 minutes
Time you will need to cook any ingredients: 20 minutes
Total Time to prepare and cook the meal: 30 minutes

Nutritional Information for one serving:
- Total Cals: 131 calories
- Protein: 7.2 grams
- Fat: 4 grams
- Fiber: 24 grams
- Carbohydrates: 18 grams

Ingredients:
- 4 cups of Rice Krispies
    - You don't have to use the name brand. Find the brand you like the most and use that, as long as it's the same type of cereal.
- 60 grams of vanilla protein powder
    - This is roughly equivalent to 2 standard sized scoops.
- ½ cup of your favorite peanut butter
- ½ cup honey

Directions:
1. Mix honey, peanut butter, and your protein powder until completely mixed with a nice, consistent texture.
2. Slowly, pour in your four cups of Rice Krispies cereal to your sticky mixture and stir.
   a. This part is going to take some effort because of how thick the mixture will become with the addition of the cereal. Keep at it and, if you need to, take a break or let someone else mix it for a bit. It uses a lot of muscle.
3. Bring out a baking pan (this recipe fits an 8x8 pan) and line it with parchment paper.
   a. You don't need to line it with paper, but it makes getting your treats out a lot easier.
4. Scoop your Sticky Rice Krispies mixture into your pan and press it down so it fills the container evenly.
5. Place the pan with the mixture in it in the refrigerator and let it sit for 20 minutes.
6. Once they've cooled and set, cut your Rice Krispies Treats into 16 bars (cut a 3x3 grid into the bars).

These are easy to store and easy to eat treats for on the go or a quiet night at home. They're easy enough to make, require very few ingredients, and don't require heat to "cook" so your kids can help you make them (or you can just have the kids mix the ingredients to tire them out and give you a break).

If you want to add a bit of decadence to your Rice Krispies Treats, feel free to melt around a quarter of a cup of dark chocolate while the treats cool and set. When they're still cool, drizzle the chocolate over top, just enough so that each bite contains a nice chocolate flavor.

Recipe 20: Crustless Pumpkin Pie

Serving Size: 1 Slice

Time you will need to prepare your ingredients: 10 minutes
Time you will need to cook any ingredients: 50 minutes
Total Time to prepare and cook the meal: 60 minutes

Nutritional Information for one serving:
- Total Cals: 169 calories
- Protein: 26 grams
- Fat: 3 grams
- Fiber: 2.3 grams
- Carbohydrates: 11 grams

Ingredients:
- 2 large eggs
- 1 ½ cups 0% fat greek yogurt (Plain, no flavor)
- 1 15 ounce can of pure pumpkin
  - Do not get this confused with pumpkin pie filling, the two are different in many ways (including calories and macro counts).
- 120 grams (4 scoops) of whey protein
  - You have some flexibility with your whey protein. You can use vanilla, chocolate, or cinnamon.
- 2 Tablespoons of pumpkin pie spice
- 1 teaspoon Natural sweetener

Directions:

1. Before you begin anything, Set your oven's dial to to 325 degrees Fahrenheit.
2. Add your dry ingredients to a large bowl (your choice of whey protein flavors, pumpkin pie spice, and sweetener). Mix a few times to get the powders combined.
3. Add your eggs to the mixture along with your can of pure pumpkin, and greek yogurt and stir all of them together. Stir until the ingredients are well combined and have a consistent texture.
4. Spray a pie pan with nonstick spray and pour your pumpkin pie mixture into it. Place the pie pan into the oven. On the lower rack, place an oven safe dish full of water to prevent the pie drying out during baking. Cook for 50 minutes.
5. Once the pie is cooked, place in your refrigerator for roughly 5 hours to cool and set.
6. Once the pie is set, cut into 6 equally sized pieces and enjoy!

Like regular pumpkin pie, you can always add whipped cream or syrup on top. It will add to your calorie and macro counts, of course, but sometimes a treat is necessary.

Recipe 21: Vanilla Birthday Cake

Serving Size: 1 Slice (⅛ of the cake)

Time you will need to prepare your ingredients: 5 minutes
Time you will need to cook any ingredients: 10 minutes
Total Time to prepare and cook the meal: 4 hours and 10 minutes

Nutritional Information for one serving:
- Total Cals: 65 calories
- Protein: 5 grams
- Fat: 1.2 gram
- Fiber: 0 grams
- Carbohydrates: 10 grams

Ingredients:
- 4 Tablespoons of Old fashioned oats
- 2 Tablespoons of quick oats
- 1 30-gram scoop of vanilla protein powder
- 8 grams of sugar free, nonfat pudding mix
- 75 grams of light Vanilla greek yogurt
- Rainbow sprinkles

Directions:

1. In a large bowl safe for microwave use (a larger one than you think you may need) pour both kinds of oats. Then fill with water so that the top layer of oats is just covered by the water.
2. Place the bowl in the microwave and cook the water and oats for a minute and a half. Once the oats are cooks, stir until most of the water has been soaked up by the oats. Once that's done, pour more water into the bowl so that the water level is equal to the oats level.
3. Place the bowl back into the microwave and cook for another minute and a half. Once that's finished, take it out and stir until the water is absorbed.
4. Add about half the water as you did the previous time and cook the oats again for another minute and a half. Take out and stir until the water is absorbed.
5. Add half the amount of water from step 4 (about ¼ the amount of the oats) and cook one last time for a minute and a half. Once that's done, stir it and make sure all the water is absorbed into the oats.
6. Add the vanilla protein powder and sugar free, nonfat pudding mix into your fully cooked oats and stir until well combined. Do this step quickly after you pull the oats from the microwave; you want them to be as warm as possible when mixing.
7. Cover the bowl in foil or cling wrap and place it into your refrigerator for 4 - 6 hours minimum. The longer you keep your oats mixture in the refrigerator, the safer you are. If you want to be the safest, keep the bowl in the refrigerator overnight.
8. After at least 4 hours, take out the oats from the refrigerator and top with the vanilla greek yogurt and sprinkle the rainbow sprinkles on top.
9. Cut the cake into eight equally sized pieces and enjoy your shameless treat!

Recipe 22: Chocolate Muffins (with Optional Caramel Coconut Icing)

Serving Size: 1 Muffin

Time you will need to prepare your ingredients: 15 minutes
Time you will need to cook any ingredients: 15 minutes
Total Time to prepare and cook the meal: 30 minutes (plus 5 minutes to cool and set)

Nutritional Information (per muffin without caramel topping):
- Total Cals: 80 calories
- Protein: 6 grams
- Fat: 2 grams
- Fiber: 0 grams
- Carbohydrates: 11 grams

Nutritional Information (per muffin with caramel topping):
- Total Cals: 143
- Protein: 6 grams
- Fat: 5 grams
- Fiber: 0 grams
- Carbohydrates: 20 grams

Ingredients for Chocolate Muffins:
- 2 scoops of chocolate whey protein powder (roughly 60 grams)
  - Vanilla whey protein powder also works well to make a more complex flavor.
- ¾ Cup all purpose flour
- 2 Tablespoon cocoa powder
- ½ teaspoon baking powder
- ½ banana
- 1 large egg
- ½ Cup almond milk
- 2 Tablespoons butter

- 1 Tablespoon low fat greek yogurt
- 1 teaspoon vanilla extract

Ingredients for Caramel Coconut Icing:
- ½ cup sugar free caramel sauce
- ½ cup shredded coconut

Directions for the Chocolate Muffins:
1. Set your oven's dial to to 350 degrees Fahrenheit.
2. In one large bowl place your whey protein powder, flour, cocoa powder, baking powder, and banana. Mix with a wooden or plastic spoon until the texture is consistent (you may have to smash the bananas a bit, so don't be afraid to put some muscle into it!).
3. In a second bowl, mix together the egg and almond milk and whisk them together. Once those two ingredients are well combined, add your softened butter, greek yogurt, and vanilla extract and mix to combine. Because the greek yogurt and butter are a bit thicker, it is much easier to mix them in one at a time.
4. Pour your dry mixture over your wet one and stir to combine into a dough. Thoroughly grease a muffin tin and fill each compartment roughly ¾ the way full. (This recipe makes a dozen muffins, so two muffin pans with six compartments each is acceptable).
5. Place your full muffin tins into your preheated oven and bake for 10 minutes.
   a. Based on your oven, your muffins may need more time to bake. It's always safer to check how well cooked your muffins are by sticking a toothpick in the top of one of the muffins. Pull the toothpick out. If some muffin sticks to the toothpick, the muffins need a bit more time. If the toothpick comes out clean, the muffins are cooked perfectly.
6. Once the muffins are done baking, pull them out and set them aside to cool down for at least 5 minutes.

Directions for the Caramel Coconut Icing:
1. In a bowl, mix together the caramel sauce and coconut shavings.
2. Once the muffins have cooled enough (at least 5 minutes), use a normal table spoon to spread 1 Tablespoon of caramel and coconut mixture onto each of your muffins

These muffins are a great treat to have any time of the year (and with any meal to give you a bit more calories and macros if one of your meals is low on either). These also work well if you are trying to help your kids eat healthier. The best part: They won't know it's healthy. When they do find out it's healthy, they'll realize how good healthy food can be and maybe start a habit of smarter eating.

Recipe 23: Chocolate Covered Nut Clusters

Serving Size: 1 Bite (makes 20 servings)

Time you will need to prepare your ingredients: 25 minutes
Time you will need to cook any ingredients: 5 minutes
Total Time to prepare and cook the meal: 30 minutes

Nutritional Information for one serving:
- Total Cals: 54
- Protein: 1 gram
- Fat: 5 grams
- Fiber: 0.5 grams
- Carbohydrates: 3 grams

Ingredients:
- 20 Almonds
- 10 Pecans
- 10 Walnuts
- 1 Package of baking chocolate
  - While any chocolate will do, dark chocolate is preferred because of how rich it is. Milk chocolate is sweet and sugary, which leads to wanting more.
- Coarse cut sea salt
  - Really, any form of sea salt will do, but coarse cut offers the texture that makes the clusters feel more complete.

Directions:

1. With a knife, half your pecans and walnuts so you have 20 halves of each.
2. To melt the chocolate, you have a few options:
   a. Use a double boiler: Boil water in a large pot and place a large metal mixing bowl over the top. Place your baking chocolate into the bowl and let the steam melt it.
   b. Use a fondue pot: Whether electronic or otherwise, use the fondue pot similar to the double boiler, or follow the directions on the device itself.
   c. Use the microwave: By far the most common and easiest method, using a microwave is as simple as placing the baking chocolate into a bowl safe for microwave use and placing it in the microwave. Heat for 30 seconds, take out of the microwave, stir, and repeat. Do this until the chocolate is smooth and fully melted.
3. Cover a surface with enough wax paper to hold all twenty clusters.
4. Once the chocolate is melted, place a nut on the prongs of a fork and dip it gently into the melted chocolate. Let it sit above the chocolate for a moment so the extra chocolate drips back into the bowl. Repeat with all of the first type of nut.
5. Move to the second type of nut and repeat the process you did with the first nut. Instead of placing this kind of nut onto the wax paper, lay it so that it's mostly on one of the nuts already on the wax paper. This will start to form the "clusters."
6. Repeat with the third type of nut.
7. While the chocolate on the final nuts is not fully cooled, sprinkle each with a light pinch of sea salt. Let sit for 15 minutes.
8. Store at room temperature, in the refrigerator, or the freezer.

These treats are perfect for a light dessert at small get-togethers or group outings. The rich taste of the dark chocolate fills up your need for a bit of decadence while the nuts give you a bit of protein to finish up any meal and finish filling you up. The salt is there to make all the flavors pop and really make the one bite serving size worth it.

Recipe 24: Flourless Chocolate Cup Cake (Not Cupcakes)

Serving Size: 1 Cup of Cake (recipes makes 8 cups)

Time you will need to prepare your ingredients: 10 minutes
Time you will need to cook any ingredients: 15 minutes
Total Time to prepare and cook the meal: 25 minutes

Nutritional Information for one serving:
- Total Cals: 136 calories
- Protein: 3 grams
- Fat: 8 grams
- Fiber: 2 grams
- Carbohydrates: 15 grams

Ingredients:
- 6 ounces of dark baking chocolate
- ¼ cup of pumpkin puree
- 1 ½ Tablespoon of real maple syrup
- 1 teaspoon of vanilla extract
- 1 Large egg
- Egg whites from 3 large eggs
- Salt

Directions:
1. Set your oven's dial to to 350 degree Fahrenheit.
2. Spray 8 oven safe mugs with nonstick spray and set onto a baking sheet.
3. Crumble the baking chocolate and place it into a large bowl safe for microwave use. Place the bowl in the microwave and cook for 30 seconds. Remove from the microwave and stir. Repeat in 30 second intervals until the chocolate is fully melted and silky smooth. Let the chocolate cool for no more than 6 minutes.
4. Once the chocolate is cooled down a bit, mix pumpkin puree into it. Next add one whole egg, maple syrup, and vanilla extract. Mix until everything is completely combined.
5. In another bowl, place the whites from three large eggs and beat until it looks like whipped cream.
6. Scrape the foamy egg whites into your chocolate pumpkin mixture and fold gently. Add a pinch of salt to the mixture as you fold.
7. Place enough batter into each cup so that it rests just about the halfway point. Place in your preheated oven for 15 minutes. Once the timer goes off, take a toothpick and stick it in the top center of one of the cup cakes. If it comes out clean, the cake is ready to be eaten.

This is another fun recipe to serve up at parties or gatherings (anything from a child's birthday party or after school hangout to a late work meeting). Not only is it a fun way to present the food, it makes sure no one gets a smaller piece, plus no cutting involved.

Feel free to add whipped cream or ice cream to the top for a slightly less healthy, but infinitely more delicious treat.

Recipe 25: Fruit Pizza

Serving Size: 1 Slice or bar (Recipe makes 30 servings)

Time you will need to prepare your ingredients: 15 minutes
Time you will need to cook any ingredients: roughly 15 minutes
Total Time to prepare and cook the meal: 30 minutes

Nutritional Information for one serving:
- Total Cals: 140 calories
- Protein: 2 grams
- Fat: 5 grams
- Fiber: 1 gram
- Carbohydrates: 24 grams

Crust Ingredients:
- 2 cups all purpose flour
- ½ teaspoon baking soda
- ⅛ teaspoon cinnamon
  - Of course, freshly ground or grated is alway better than pre ground.
- ⅔ cups granulated sugar
- ⅔ cups light brown sugar
- ¼ cup unsalted butter
- The whites from 2 large eggs
- ¼ cup apple sauce (unsweetened is preferred)
- 2 teaspoons of vanilla extract
- ⅔ cup white chocolate chips
  - You can also use bars or baking white chocolate if you crumple them (not grind because you want that extra texture).
  - You can also substitute this for dark or milk chocolate chips or crumples. Chocolate and fruit is a common and so delicious combination.
- Salt

Frosting Ingredients:
- 8 ounces fat free cream cheese
- ½ cup confectioners or powdered sugar
- 1 teaspoon vanilla extract

Fruits:
- 3 kiwi
- 8 - 10 strawberries
- 1 cup of blueberries
- 1 cup of raspberries
- 1 cup of blackberries

Crust Directions:
1. Set your oven's dial to to 350 degrees Fahrenheit.
2. Pull out a baking pan or 2 pie pans and spray them down with non stick spray. Set those aside. Soften the butter in the microwave (do not melt).
3. In a large sized mixing bowl, whisk together the softened butter, egg whites, applesauce, and vanilla extract. The mixture should get fluffy after a few minutes of quick whisking.
4. In a separate, medium sized mixing bowl, mix the flour, baking soda, cinnamon, and a pinch of salt until everything is evenly combined.
5. Pour the contents of the medium sized mixing bowl (the flour, baking soda, cinnamon, etc) into the large mixing bowl containing your eggs and butter mixture. Gently fold the wet and dry ingredients together with a rubber spatula or plastic spoon. Mix until the ingredients form a smooth batter (you may need to add water).
6. Once your batter is smooth, gently fold the white chocolate chips or crumbles in.
7. Transfer your batter into either your baking pan or pie pans and press down using the bottom of a cup or another flat surface (you want it as even as possible so it cooks evenly -- although raw cookie does is delicious).

8. Bake your crust for around 15 minutes. You'll know it's finished when the edges are browning and you can stick the center with a toothpick and pull it out clean.
9. Once baked, remove the crust from the oven and let cool either on a wire rack or a newspaper.

Frosting Directions:
1. In a large mixing bowl, beat the cream cheese (this is easy with an electric mixer or power mixer). Slowly mix in the confectioners or powdered sugar and vanilla extract into the cream cheese. Don't stop the mixer if using an electric one, but do turn it down so sugar doesn't explode all over your kitchen.

Assembling your Fruit Pizza:
1. Cut your crust into 30 bars (this is easily accomplished by cutting two lines one way and four the other for a total of 15 bars, then cutting each of these bars in half).
2. Spread around a tablespoon to a tablespoon and a half of frosting on each bar.
3. Cut your strawberries and kiwi into small pieces and organize the fruits one each cookie however you see fit. Place in the fridge to store for up to two days.

This is, in my opinion, an underrated dessert regardless of any diets. It's commonly made in middle and high school cooking classes, but soon after forgotten about completely. Why is it forgotten so easily? I have no idea, but it deserves to be present in more lives.

It combines your desires for sweets (by the cookie crust) and your favorite fruits, which you can add or remove to the recipe as you see fit. It's perfect for a large group of people who all like different fruits and combinations of fruits.

Chapter 5: Small Meals, Snacks, and Sides

These recipes are designed specifically to either augment a meal to help meet your goals, or are here for you to sneak away from your desk in the middle of the day to grab something small to eat to keep your stomach from growling too loudly.

Recipe 26: Bacon Cheddar Ranch Cauliflower Salad

Serving Size: 1 Cup

Time you will need to prepare your ingredients: 10 minutes
Time you will need to cook any ingredients: 10 minutes
Total Time to prepare and cook the meal: 20 minutes

Nutritional Information for one serving:
- Total Cals: 210 calories
- Protein: 19 grams
- Fat: 7 grams
- Fiber: 14 grams
- Carbohydrates: 19 grams

Ingredients:
- 6 cups of cauliflower
- ¼ cup cheddar cheese
- 2 slices of bacon
- ½ cup fat free greek yogurt
- 2 Tablespoons of ranch seasoning (roughly one packet)
- Pepper and salt

Directions:

1. Chop cauliflower into florets (the end most pieces of the plant). Smaller pieces will provide a more consistent texture, but big pieces will offer bite sized morsels for you to chew on. Place the cut cauliflower into a large pot.
2. Pour water into the pot so that the tops of the cauliflower are covered.
3. Set your stove top for high heat and let the water reach a boil. Let the cauliflower boil until tender, which is usually around 7 minutes.
   a. Cook time will vary based on the size of the pot and your personal stove top. It can be anywhere from 5 minutes to 10 minutes. Check occasionally by pulling a piece of cauliflower from the water (with tongs or a spoon) and feeling it. If it's not tender, place it back and check in a minute or so.
4. Once the cauliflower is tender, drain it using a strainer and set that aside to cool.
5. In a large sized bowl, mix together your fat free greek yogurt, ranch seasoning, and Pepper and salt. Pour your cauliflower into the bowl with your greek yogurt mixture and stir to combine until every piece of cauliflower is coated with the greek yogurt. Set aside.
6. In a pan, cook your slices of bacon until they are crispy. Place the cooked bacon on a paper towel lined plate to soak up some of the excess fat.
7. When they meat is cool enough, crumble it over the cauliflower along with the shredded cheese. Mix the ingredients together just enough so the bacon and cheese is spread throughout the dish and enjoy!

This is a great recipe for any occasion. People do tend to give you a look like "you brought cauliflower to a picnic?" That look vanishes as soon as they take their first bite into something they never thought could be so delicious.

Recipe 27: Orange Coconut Bars

Serving Size: 1 Bar

Time you will need to prepare your ingredients: 20 minutes
Time you will need to cook any ingredients: 20 minutes
Total Time to prepare and cook the meal: 40 minutes (plus overnight!)

Nutritional Information for one serving:
- Total Cals: 242 calories
- Protein: 3.3 grams
- Fat: 17.5 grams
- Fiber: 0.5 grams
- Carbohydrates: 19.2 grams

Crust Ingredients:
- ⅓ Cups of coconut oil
  - A helpful hint regarding Coconut oil: If you want a stronger coconut flavor in your food, use unrefined coconut oil. If you want a less noticeable coconut flavor, use refined coconut oil.
- 3 Tablespoon maple syrup
- ¾ cups coconut flour

Filling Ingredients:
- 4 large eggs
- 4 large eggs' yolks
- ⅔ Cups of honey
- 1 Cup orange juice (fresh is always better)
- 2 Tablespoons of orange zest
- ⅔ Cups of coconut oil
- 3 Tablespoon shredded coconut
- Salt

Directions:
1. Before anything else, preheat the oven to 350 degrees Fahrenheit. Take out an 8x8 baking dish and lightly coat the inside with coconut oil. Line the dish with baking paper (it should stick to the sides due to the coconut oil).

2. Soften your coconut oil for your crust in the microwave for about 5 seconds. In a medium sized bowl, place your softened coconut oil and the maple syrup. Using a hand mixer, cream the two ingredients together until they are well combined and fluffy.
3. Slowly stir in the coconut flour, being careful not to add too much or stir too fast, until it solidifies into a dough.
4. Transfer your dough into the baking dish and, using your hands, spread the dough out so that it covers all parts of the pan as evenly as possible. Place what will become the crust into the preheated oven and bake until the center area is golden and the edges are golden brown (roughly 8 to 10 minutes). Once cooked, remove and set aside to cool.
5. In a medium pot, throw together all of your eggs (the eggs and the egg yolks) . honey, orange juice, orange zest, and a very small pinch of salt. Whisk the ingredients together until combined. Turn the heat on your stove top to medium-low.
6. As your mixture warms up, add your coconut oil and whisk constantly until your mixture thickens (it should take about 8 minutes).
7. Make sure your crust is cooled down (it can be warmed than room temperature, but shouldn't be hot to the touch). If your crust is cool enough, pour the filling over it and spread evenly using a spatula or spoon. If you can't get into every corner, shake the baking dish with small, quick shakes to spread your filling in all the hard to reach places.
8. Let your bars rest on the counter for about half an hour then transfer the to the refrigerator overnight (this step is crucial! -- Let your bars rest in the chill chest for at least 8 hours before attempting to cut and serve).
9. Once they've set and cooled enough, pull your bars out and transfer them to a cutting board (using the baking paper underneath to gently remove them from the baking dish). Sprinkle the block with shredded coconut and cut into 16 evenly sized squares.
10. If you aren't going to eat them all right away, return the uneaten ones to the refrigerator to maintain their shape.

Recipe 28: Cranberry Sauce with Pears

Serving Size: Roughly ¼ of a cup (Recipes makes 13 servings)

Time you will need to prepare your ingredients: 5 minutes
Time you will need to cook any ingredients: 15 minutes
Total Time to prepare and cook the meal: 20 minutes

Nutritional Information for one serving:
- Total Cals: 61
- Protein: 0 gram
- Fat: 0 grams
- Fiber: 2 grams
- Carbohydrates: 16 grams

Ingredients:
- 12 ounce cranberries
- 2 pears
- ½ cup honey
- Water

Directions:
1. Peel the pears, remove the core, and cut into small ½ inch cubes.
2. In a medium pot over high heat, bring roughly a cup and a half of water to a boil.
3. When the water starts to boil, place your cubed pears, cranberries, and honey into the pot and give the whole thing a few stirs.
4. Once the mixture hits a rolling boil, reduce the heat to medium to medium low and simmer for roughly 15 minutes.
   a. A good way to check how close the mixture is to being cooked is the cranberries. If the skin breaks on the cranberries and the insides burst, your sauce is close to being finished.
5. Once done, remove the pot from the heat and let it rest at room temperature for at least 15 minutes. Once the sauce is close to room temperature, place it in the refrigerator and let it chill for an hour.

If you're tired of the same old cranberry sauce for the holidays, surprise people by making this unique flavor experience. Your guests won't know what hit them when they were expecting the same cranberry sauce they've been eating since they were children.

Recipe 29: Oatmeal Cookies with White Chocolate Frosting

Serving Size: 2 cookies (Recipe makes 23 cookies)

Time you will need to prepare your ingredients: 10 minutes
Time you will need to cook any ingredients: 10 minutes
Total Time to prepare and cook the meal: 20 minutes

Nutritional Information for one serving:
- Total Cals: 84 calories
- Protein: 1 gram
- Fat: 5 grams
- Fiber: 0 grams
- Carbohydrates: 13 grams

Ingredients:
- ½ cup of all-purpose flour
- ½ cup of sugar
- ½ teaspoon of cinnamon
- ⅓ teaspoon of baking powder
- ½ cup of oats
- ¼ cup of unsalted butter
- 2 Tablespoons of milk
    - This recipe uses 1% milk. Skim milk will work, technically, but will not provide the same texture as 1% milk.
- 2 Tablespoons of honey
- 1 teaspoon of vanilla extract
- 4 ounces of white baking chocolate
    - You can also use dark or milk chocolate, but it will slightly affect the calories and macros count.
- Salt

Cookie Directions:
1. Preheat you oven to 375 degrees Fahrenheit.
2. In a medium sized mixing bowl, pour the flour, granulated sugar, cinnamon, baking powder, salt, and oats. Mix the ingredients until they are well combined and set to the side for the time being.
3. Place the butter into a bowl safe for microwave use and microwave for 30 to 45 seconds until completely melted.
4. In a large mixing bowl, pour melted butter, 1% milk, honey, and vanilla extract. Use an electric or power mixer to combine the ingredients (you can do this by hand but it will take much longer and much more muscle).
5. Turn the electric mixer down to slow speeds and slowly pour one fourth of your dry ingredients into the bowl. After each pour, let the mixer combine the ingredients before adding the next fourth.
6. Using a teaspoon, scoop the batter onto a series of baking sheets lined with baking paper.
7. Bake the cookies for 7 - 9 minutes or until golden brown. Remove the baking sheets from the oven and let the cookies set and cool on the m for at least a minute and a half. Once the batter has set, move the cookies to a wire rack or a newspaper to continue cooling.

Frosting Directions:
1. Place the chocolate chips or baking chocolate into a bowl safe for microwave use and microwave for 30 - 45 seconds. Remove the chocolate from the microwave and stir. Return the chocolate to the microwave and repeat until the chocolate is fully melted and smooth.
2. Once the cookies are cooled fully, dip up to one half of each cookie into the chocolate and return to the original baking sheets lined with paper to set.

These cookies will be thinner than most people are used to, but that's what allows a serving to be 2 cookies, instead of 1. These are great for parties or get-togethers to have out for people to eat throughout the night and enjoy. Little will they know that they'll be eating some of the healthiest cookies they've ever had.

Recipe 30: Chia Coconut Pudding with Raspberries

Serving Size: 1 cup (recipe makes 2 servings)

Time you will need to prepare your ingredients: 15 minutes
Time you will need to cook any ingredients: 0 minutes
Total Time to prepare and cook the meal: 15 minutes plus one night in the refrigerator to cool.

Nutritional Information for one serving:
- Total Cals: 157 calories
- Protein: 4 grams
- Fat: 10 grams
- Fiber: 10 grams
- Carbohydrates: 15 grams

Ingredients:
- 1 cup of fresh raspberries
- ½ cup of coconut milk
- ½ cup almond milk
- 2 Tablespoons of Chia seeds
- 1 Tablespoon of shredded coconut
- 1 Tablespoon of honey
- 1 teaspoon of lime juice
- 1 teaspoon of zest from a lime

Directions:
1. In a large mixing bowl, pour half of the raspberries (½ cups). Pour the coconut milk, almond milk, chia seeds, shredded coconut, honey lime juice, and lime zest over the raspberries and gently fold the ingredients together.
2. Once the dry and wet ingredients begin to come together, switch it up and start to mix the ingredients with more vigor until well combined.
3. Transfer the contents from the large mixing bowl into a sealable container (a large tupperware container works well). Seal the container and move to the refrigerator. Let the pudding sit over night (or at least 7 hours if you're making this in the morning).
4. Scoop half the pudding into a dish and top with half of the remaining raspberries.

On those hot summer days, you may want to dive into a nice bowl of ice cream to help quell the heat (especially when you hear the ice cream truck jingling down the road). This recipe is made to help prevent those temptations by giving you something nearly as sweet as ice cream, and much healthier for you.

While the texture and looks of this pudding can be off putting to some, once they try it they won't want to have just one bite. If the person in question still refuses to try this treat, you can always make it without the chia seeds (or just say shucks to them and enjoy their pudding as well!).

Recipe 31: Classic (Flourless) Brownies

Serving Size: 1 bar (recipe makes 12 servings)

Time you will need to prepare your ingredients: 10 minutes
Time you will need to cook any ingredients: 30 minutes
Total Time to prepare and cook the meal: 40 minutes

Nutritional Information for one serving:
- Total Cals: 131 calories
- Protein: 6 grams
- Fat: 5 grams
- Fiber: 3 grams
- Carbohydrates: 26 grams

Ingredients:
- 1 large egg
- The whites from 1 large egg
- ½ cups of cocoa powder
- 1 teaspoon of baking soda
- ½ cups of water
- ½ cups of honey
- 1 teaspoon vanilla extract
- ¾ cups of chocolate chips
  - While Sweet milk chocolate chips are certainly delicious, dark chocolate chips are much more decadent. White chocolate chips will also add a nice flavor to the chocolate brownies. Use whichever chocolate chips you prefer, or a combination of all three.

Dilons:

Preheat the oven to 325 degrees Fahrenheit.

In a small mixing bowl, whisk the egg and egg whites until smooth.

. In a larger sized mixing bowl, mix the cocoa powder, salt, and baking soda. Once the powders are fully combined, add the egg mixture and stir to combine.

4. Pour the water into the mixture and a few times. Once the powder and water is loosely mixed, add the honey and vanilla extract until everything is completely combined. Once all of the lumps have been smoothed out, gently fold whichever chocolate chips you decided on into the batter.

5. Pull a 9x9 baking pan out and pour the batter into it so it fills the bottom.

6. Set the batter into the oven and bake for around 30 minutes. You can check if it's finished by sticking a toothpick in the center of the top of the brownies. If it comes out clean, the brownies are finished.

7. Allow the brownies to cool for at least ten minutes before cutting into 12 bars.

Not all foods can be fun and innovative. Sometimes you just want one of the classic desserts. These brownies, while modified to be healthier and gluten free, are as close as you can get to the classic food without putting your diet in jeopardy.

Conclusion

Thank you again for picking up and reading "Flexible Dieting and IIFYM Cookbook: 31 High Protein Recipes to Help You Lose Fat and Build Muscle." I hope you found at least a few recipes you are willing to try, and I hope you enjoyed learning about all of these delicious and healthy alternatives to your everyday meals.

CPSIA information can be obtained
at www.ICGtesting.com
Printed in the USA
BVOW06s1832230417
482050BV00008B/189/P